Mount Kurama and the Emerald Lake
Child and Youth Reiki Program

Mythological Reiki Tales
Empowering Kids! With Resources for Parents, Educators and Reiki Teachers

Cheryl Jiala Driskell

Cover Design
Amanda DeVries Graphics Design Services
www.amandadevries.com

Dedication

...For little star who has guided me through my own mountain gates to greater understandings and surrender...

Contents

Acknowledgments

It is with great gratitude that I thank the one loving source and all of its loving manifestations for the continued guidance in all that I do. Without the support of generous Reiki teachers such as Leah Smith and Louise Jackson I would not have witnessed the beauty of Reiki. Thank you also to my other teachers Shirley King, Lorie Carson, Sabina Wasserlauf, Inayat and Harry Boehm (posthumously) for additional guidance, insights, love and understanding.

The wonders of my life have been shared with many loving beings and each of them has offered me many opportunities to know myself and the universe in all its beauty. Thank you to my parents Carole and Ernie, grandmothers Evelyn and Alice, Rob, Chelsea, Megan, Garth, Lisa, Janet, Bob, Jane I. (Pepper), Marie, Tamara, Catherine, Gene, Johanne, Alan (teddy bear), Francine, Nathalie, Ashley, James, Shawn, Diane, Victor, Dylan, Jessie, Pauline, Maureen, Sheri, Kyle, Mary, Paul, Helen, Tom, Evalisa, Lauren, Amy, the two Suzannes, Andrée (swamp woman), Jeannine, Stéphane, Jane M., Lyne, the two Donnas, Ed, Virginia, my wonderful students and clients, as well as so many more for their generosity of spirit and many forms of guidance and support.

Thank you Amanda for your inspired cover art! With gratitude to Sigrid Macdonald for her sincere assistance with the editorial and final preparatory process of this book, and for the kindness, encouragement, love and grace of my dear friend, Tara, in all of her light.

Commonly Asked Questions

What is Reiki?

Reiki is a wonderful, non-invasive, hands-on, self-loving and self-care tool. The "Rei" has been considered to mean "universal." It has also been interpreted as "higher knowledge" (1) or "consciousness." The "Ki" is the life force energy as in "Chi" or "Prana." Therefore, Reiki is the experience of life force energy being consciously guided through the body.

The individual practicing Reiki is the channel of this energy, welcoming the Reiki, offering love and ultimate health for their "self" or another. Reiki is used with the intention that it offers the highest good for the individual/s involved. It has the effect of assisting both the individual offering the Reiki as it flows through them and the person receiving the Reiki.

Reiki is not a religion and can be considered a philosophy that supports the individual development experience. It fosters self-understanding and personal acceptance, and nurtures the loving and compassionate heart to greater opening.

How can Reiki help my child or someone else?

Reiki has an immediate calming effect. It would seem to assist individuals in signaling their parasympathetic nervous system, allowing a whole host of calming benefits, including a lessening of anxiety and overall stress. It has been noted to provide balancing and health to any part of the body, mind and spirit. It can be used for hyperactivity, difficulty focusing, cuts, burns, emergencies such as shock or other trauma, or for chronic illness, stress, fatigue, anxiety, emotional or psychological discomfort and more.

Reiki assists individuals in finding balance in their life. A child who has been regularly in a hyper state may become more at peace and better able to focus on everyday matters. Or children who are generally ill at ease in their bodies may become more comfortable. It also has the power of opening the young person to self-empowerment, taking charge of their own wellness and seeing how they can effect change in their own lives. This program is designed to enable the young person to connect specific self-affirming statements (affirmations) to their Reiki experience. They can therefore help their minds to develop and maintain positive thought processes, which will assist them in the creation of a positive and loving view of "self." In this way the long-term benefits will be immeasurable!

Can Reiki harm my child?

A well received energy healer and teacher of mine has noted that a child's Chakras (vortexes of spinning energy supplying our body with necessary energy) are smaller than an adults and as such should not be exposed to too much energy at any one time. This is said to be true also for elderly people, whose Chakras have become smaller as they have aged and similarly true for seriously ill people whose chakras are in a diminished capacity. (2)

Although Reiki teachers are generally taught that the "Rei" is an intelligent energy and knows the place and amount of energy to accommodate a healing, I would just ask that you note this word of caution. It may be most appropriate to tell your children that they only need practise Reiki upon themselves or others for three to five minutes at a time.

Where does Reiki come from?

The Reiki taught today by Western Reiki teachers has tended to come from the school of thought and experience, originally taught by a Japanese gentleman named Dr. Mikao Usui. He was said to have been meditating upon Mount Kurama in Japan, when he received the process of welcoming in the Reiki energy, and the associated symbols and teachings. He passed his new understandings along to a select few students, who over time passed it along to numerous individuals, to assist many with their well-being.

There have been numerous traditions or philosophies throughout the centuries that have supported the process of hands-on self-care or healing. Reiki has been noted as being similar to other such processes previously shared and practised in some Buddhist communities in Japan, and in other spiritual communities around the world, with the process offered under different names.

Are there other levels of Reiki and can my child take them?

Reiki generally consists of four education levels. For this program, the children are learning the basics of level one, but with less history and fewer hand positions. Level two is often practised to deepen the experience of the flow of the Reiki, and includes learning three symbols that assist in this process, as well as offering the opportunity to begin distance healing. Those individuals who wish to professionally practise or teach Reiki take levels three and four.

Children who wish to enhance their understanding and experience of Reiki may wish to approach a teacher when they are 14 to16 years of age, and receive their adult level one training at this time. Once they have completed level one, they can continue on thereafter, depending upon their maturity and respect for the processes they are being taught. A Reiki teacher would ask them to seriously consider the steps they are taking before offering them further teaching.

Program Essentials

The Creation of Mount Kurama and The Emerald Lake

Mount Kurama and the Emerald Lake was created to empower young people. A number of my adult students stated how wonderful it would be to have their children take a Reiki course. They wanted their children to reap the same benefits that they were now experiencing. So, of course, I looked for one! But, sadly, I couldn't find one that offered a step-by-step process for Reiki teachers, educators and parents to share with their children/students.

After some time, I thought perhaps it would be exciting for me to develop a program. I'm not much for leaving things undone. So, I began the development of a mythological Reiki tale for children and youth. Through this they could explore Reiki for the first time. Why not make it fun and accessible while showing the great value of Reiki in their lives!

There are two stories: one for younger children and then the original tale intended for those over ten years of age. Even adults can gather awakenings from either story. Insight is never wasted or lost. Having been awakened in us once, it is more easily accessible thereafter.

The stories engage the mind of the reader through the use of Reiki philosophy, universal laws, quantum physics, philosophy, teachings related to chakras, auras, and the universal rays of light, all simply imparted in the form of a mythological tale. The stories are a combination of many ideas absorbed over the years from various teachings. Each area is touched upon briefly, so as to keep it light and to encourage readers to later explore the concepts on their own, allowing their greatest potential to be expanded.

A Program to be offered by Parents, Educators and Reiki Teachers

This Reiki Program can be utilized in groups of children with a Reiki teacher or educator, or can be completed at home with one's child or children. Only Reiki teachers generally teach Reiki. As a Reiki teacher myself, I can understand the value of this process. However, I am also an Intuitive Energy Healer and as such I have seen energy moved by individuals merely by thinking a positive thought.

"It has been discovered in quantum physics that an observer's point of view determines what is seen," and therefore experienced. (3)   I have seen the "Ki" energy consciously increased and directed to various areas of discomfort in the body by those who believed this could occur, reinforcing the value of right intention.

I have also seen how wonderful young people feel when they are having a new experience/awakening and believe that they now have the power to make changes in their own body, or emotional self, and can then alter their feelings and physical sensations. How wonderful to be a part of something so possible, and ultimately so empowering!

As such, I believe that in order to reach the countless children who might not be able or wanting to participate in a class of students, a parent can simply tell a story and then share an experiment with their child, coming from the Emerald Lake water (explained further). They can then encourage their child to practise with the new Emerald energy, using their hands on their self, both during good times and when they feel unwell or sad. The child will also have the opportunity to help others in ways they could not before. This will inspire a sense of being a part of something bigger than they had known before, and participating in a process through which they can also have the experience of giving.

I spent almost nine years working for an anxiety disorders association, and have heard countless concerns from parents whose children became overwhelmed either in a classroom or just out of the blue. Imagine children who then have a connection to the Emerald Lake energy, which they can now experience merely by placing their hands face down somewhere on their bodies, with a focus on bringing in the Reiki (Emerald energy).

This would not only give a young person the courage to remain in class, but their minds would become focused, preventing the uncomfortable thoughts from arising. This is the gift. As those of us who have meditated for years know, one-pointedness, or clarity of focus, is the key to calming and balance.

How to Use the Stories

In a class situation, the stories can be broken up to ask questions and take breaks. They would otherwise be too long for the young person to absorb. Inquiry also leads to insight. Consequently, there is additional value in asking questions and taking the process more slowly. The youth program, which includes the longer story, can be offered in as little as two hours in a classroom setting, with more time necessary if there is a lot of talk and enthusiasm. The younger child program would likely take even less time, as the story is significantly shorter and there are fewer hand positions.

A parent may wish to read the story over a number of evening bedtime story sessions, asking questions and absorbing themselves in the story with their child. After reading the shorter story to a child, over a period of a year or so, the child may be ready for the longer story and the additional hand positions.

Teaching the Reiki Healing Hand Positions

At the end of each story is a page or two that includes the Reiki hand positions used for providing the hands-on self-care. I have included only seven hand positions for the older children's personal care and two for the younger child's personal care. There are three positions to offer others for the older children and one for the younger ones. Please feel free to teach as many hand positions as you believe your child/student could benefit from. In adult Reiki there are as many as 28 hand positions, used above or on the body. The child or youth may over time find that they are most comfortable with certain hand positions and not others. Ultimately, it is less important where the hands are placed as Reiki is said to go where it feels the body, mind, heart and spirit needs it to go.

You can explain the hand positions to your child/student as the way in which Lolly carried the Emerald energy back to her father. Having fallen into the Emerald Lake to attain this energy, it could simply be noted as the "Emerald energy." You could also call it "Reiki" and explain the adult awareness of this energy to your child/student.

Each hand position is associated with a self-affirming statement (affirmation). This is intended to make it easier to remember the hand position as well as to inspire some positive, affirming self-talk that may enliven a wonderful sense of self at your child's/student's deepest core. It offers the greater potential of exposing the abundance of their authentic selves as they explore life in all of its many wonders and obstacles. The affirmations also include an awareness of the "self" as the "I am", a philosophical understanding that has conscious and unconscious value throughout our external and internal journey.

The positions that can be used on others were included because they are simple, easy to remember and age appropriate. Ultimately, a Reiki teacher, educator or parent may wish to share all the commonly used Reiki hand positions with their child or students. These can be found in adult Reiki books.

The Attunement Process

Reiki Teachers

There are so many different approaches to Reiki being taught these days. Given that there are countless individuals having wonderful experiences through the many different perspectives, it is ultimately the intention that allows the individual to open to the experience of Reiki.

It is important to note this intention in the offering of attunements to the students of the Mount Kurama and the Emerald Lake Reiki Program. For this program, a teacher will be able to attune a whole room full of young students easily by first attuning a large bowl of water from the *"**Emerald Lake.**"* The water can be clear or contain green food colouring within. The children can then each place their hands gently into the water for their attunement. As in the story, they will be able to connect to the water and through this know that they have received the supportive potential of the Emerald energy (Reiki), just like our character, Lolly!

Once the child's' hands are in the water, merely ask them to say, either, "I welcome the Reiki from the Emerald Lake to flow through me", or "I welcome the Emerald energy to flow through me." Or simply have them say, "I welcome the Reiki to flow." And it will! It has already been experienced.

Parents and Educators

With right intention, anything becomes possible. The final messages of the longer story are that the past, present and future can exist in the same moment and that we are all connected by one great sea. As such, the Reiki, or the Emerald energy of the Emerald Lake is available to each of us in any moment.

The ability to use the Reiki is generally passed along from person to person through an attunement process.   An attunement is the process of preparing the person involved to receive the Reiki easily through their body. It is the welcoming of a new openness acquired through a short ritual which is generally passed from teacher to student.

If you don't have a teacher to attune your child, you can create an Emerald Lake of your own with water and green food colouring. Then, set the intention that the water be attuned with the Reiki by placing your hands in the water, and ask that the Reiki be strong and present for all individuals wanting to invite this loving energy through them.

With your intention and the open mind and spirit of your child, there is no reason that the Reiki should not become available. Indeed, it is a part of the whole through which we are all connected and therefore always available to be experienced; we only need to ask!

My Dream

Please note that my dream for this program is that it be offered for free or for a nominal fee or small donation. It is my hope that it be offered out of caring and concern for a community in need of sharing the Reiki to foster a loving universe. I hope you will enjoy this journey with your child or students. Please feel free to e-mail your thoughts or questions to contact@jiala.ca, or enter my website at www.jiala.ca. Best Wishes!

Questions for Reinforcement and Insights

These two sections are at the end of the book. The questions have been placed in order of each story's development and can be asked as you read along with the child or at the end of the story. The insight section will assist you and the child in knowing some of the underlying messages or lessons that are within the stories.

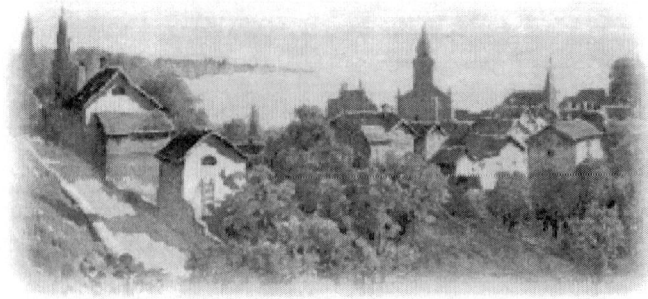

Mount Kurama and the Emerald Lake
9 years of age and under

When I would look out the window of my tower room, I could see over the whole city of Crickmore. The Tower was as bright and big as a lighthouse. The windows of the tower glittered with the sun as it poured in everyday, in everyway.

I begged my mother not to put up curtains. I wanted to see and know everything that was going on around me. So instead, we hung huge pieces of cloth in upside-down rainbow shapes all along the walls, joining one to another, all connected above and below my huge windows. There was bright red, yellow, orange, purple, blue, green and a really brilliant indigo.

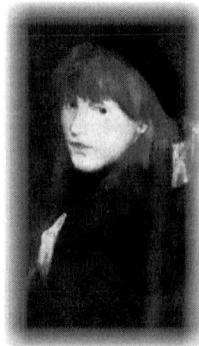

My little brother Garin called me Lolly, because he had trouble saying Lillian. I am now 11, but he was only 3 at the time, so I forgave him. The new nickname stuck and I was from thereon Lolly to everyone, young and old. Even my father thought it was the funniest name. He would call me into the parlour by yelling out, "Ooohhhh Miss Lolly, Polly, Dolly. Would you please come down here for a moment?   I'm wondering if you would

All throughout our time in the sky, I imagined that I was a wonderfully coloured bird, floating high and freely among the clouds. From time to time I could almost feel the clouds brushing against me. I felt so free up there!

We slept through the night and by the time we awoke, Garin and I could see land. It was beautiful. Japan seemed to be an amazing country. Then suddenly I saw my father's balloon begin to drop quickly from the sky. I could hear Sara's screams and my heart began to race as fast as the train that we had taken on a part of our travels.

I yelled out to Chin, "Follow that balloon!" and down we went too, though not as quickly. I suddenly saw a very large mountain ahead. It seemed to be covered by countless large green trees. It was here, at the foot of this mountain, where my father's balloon had its crash landing.

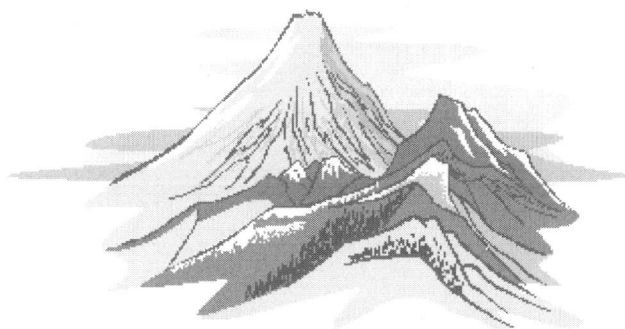

I heard a loud *WOOSH,* as they suddenly landed in a clear area of tall grasses, just in front of the mountain. I heard a scream from Sara as the balloon landed and fell over, flattening into the grasses.

My heart stopped beating for a moment and I wanted to get to them as soon as I could. By the time we landed we were still at least 150 meters or more from the other balloon. I jumped out quickly and ran with all my strength. I put my long giraffe legs into action!

When I got to the balloon I could hear nothing but a little whimper from Mr. Rickert. I noticed that the basket had landed in water! What a relief! They had been given more of a cushy landing than I believed was possible from where they fell. I was finally able to look into the basket where I saw Mr. Rickert licking my father's face!

I overheard Garin ask our pilot if any of us had done something wrong to make the wind God angry with us. Our pilot told Garin that the wind God blew us to the right place at the right time. We could have had a much harder landing.

Garin seemed relieved to hear this answer and wandered over to Mr. Rickert. I sat next to my father and asked him to wake up. But he didn't move. Sara began to cry.

I then heard our pilot telling Garin that this mountain before us was Mount Kurama. It was a special mountain. On the mountain was a wonderful garden, and if you believed the messages that could be discovered as you walked up the mountain, then you could get through the five gates that protected the garden. Inside the garden there was something really special that could help people when they were not well.

"Ah ha!" I said out loud. I knew what I was going to do. If there were ever a time to use my climbing skills, it was now. The sky was becoming red and a lot of time had seemed to pass. The sun was slowly going down.

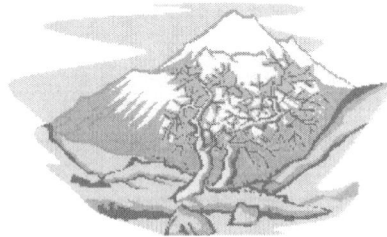

I leapt up and began to run towards the mountain. No one seemed to notice that I was leaving, so I kept on running. Then, suddenly I realized that Mr. Rickert was trying hard to keep up with me. He was quite old and tended to lay around a lot, but he wouldn't want me to go out on my own.

I had been taught to leave marks on trees in order to remember where I had been, so I could always get home. I picked up a red stone and began to mark the trees in order to find my way home.

I could feel that I knew exactly where to go. I had no doubt, even when we came in front of the first locked gate. It had been hidden behind several tall trees, but I had seen a glitter of gold that had gotten my attention.

"Mr. Rickert," I said. "Where do you think the message is hidden that I am to believe in order to get through the gate?" He gazed at me and twisted his head with some concern. Then he barked!

As if knowing what he was trying to tell me, I looked at him and said, "Yes, Mr. Rickert, there is no reason to worry. We will find our way through!"

Then, out of the blue, I heard a click followed by a loud creaking sound, as the gate suddenly opened on its own. "That's it, Mr. Rickert! **I need only believe that there is no reason to worry** and we can get through the gate."

Mr. Rickert jumped up and was the first to run through the gate. We were both very excited now! There were only four more gates to find and get through!

About 10 metres on the other side of the gate, we hit a huge piece of the mountain, like a large wall that we could most certainly not climb.

"Now, what are were we going to do?" I thought. Angrily, I threw my hands up in the air. As they were falling I hit a tree branch, upon which had been a loose stick that had now fallen to the ground.

As I picked up this stick, I saw the words carved into it, **"Just for now do not anger."**

"Mr. Rickert. Look! Here is the second message!" I was so excited that I had forgotten for that moment to be angry, and the gate seemed to joyfully swing open for us.

"Wonderful," I said aloud, so thankful for this help! Then, as we were making our way through the second gate, I heard what sounded like another gate ahead, swinging open.

"Mr. Rickert," I gasped. "What do you think is going on? Was it because I said that I was thankful that another gate opened?"

As we approached this open gate, I noticed a piece of paper stuck under a rock. There was the message!

"Just for now be thankful!"

How marvelous! I was right. I only needed to show how thankful I was for this to make my way through the third gate.

"Well, Mr. Rickert. What do you say? Shall we continue?" I was rubbing his ears now as he looked up at me quite happily. He barked as though saying *yes* to what I had asked.

This time, we seemed to be led along a winding path. It was not very wide and there were ledges with mud, tree roots and countless different types of green plants. If we were to fall, we would have a long way down to go!

Having learned the lesson of the first message, I wasn't worried. I knew we could do this, but also that we would have to work hard to get to the next gate.

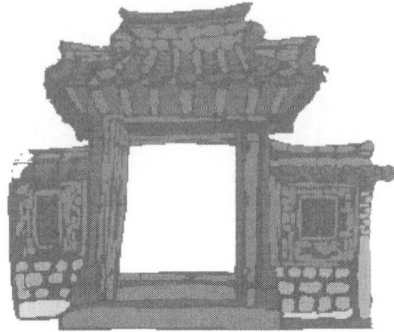

I could see now that the path was coming to an end. All at once, we seemed to have come upon a small little building with a red roof. It was right in the middle of the mountain. How fascinating! There were little stone statues out front, perhaps as many as 30 or more. They all had pleasant faces with big smiles engraved on them!

"Wait 'til I tell Father about these," I thought.

The gate that had blocked the opening to this building was wide open! "Could someone be inside," I thought.

"Come along, Mr. Rickert," I yelled as he was looking closely at the sculptures, perhaps afraid that they might move.

But he continued to bark! There in the hand of one of the statues was a piece of cloth. Upon this cloth was written the fourth message.

"Just for now work hard."

"Have we ever!" I said happily to Mr. Rickert.

"How marvelous that what I believe is opening all of these gates! It is as though each time I think or say something; I am preparing the way for the next gate to open." I paused.

"Mr. Rickert, shall we go through now, then?" I asked joyfully, as I quickly gave a loving tug to his tail. He leapt up quickly and ran immediately through the gate where he began to bark very loudly.

Running in behind him I saw now why he was barking so loudly. Before us was a huge cave that this little building and the gate had guarded. I had always been afraid of the dark, but now was the time to face that fear. I knew now that working hard had opened this gate and it would get us through to wherever the cave led.

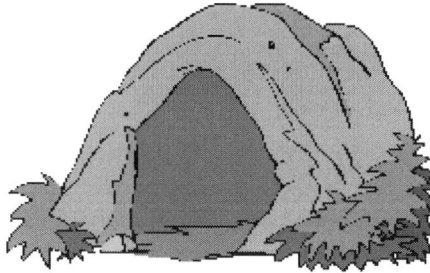

Mr. Rickert and I slowly walked into the cave that was so dark I could barely see my own hands. As we were further into the cave, I could feel that there were stringy things hanging from the ceiling.

"How yucky is this, Mr. Rickert!" I said as I walked along.

"Hey!" I suddenly yelled. "Light. There's light down there..." I started to run! Then, just as I was reaching the end of the cave, nearing the light, I tripped and fell onto my knees.

"Ooohhhh," I yelped. "That was smart, wasn't it? Running in the dark!" Then I started to laugh!

"Mr. Rickert, it's a good thing I have you with me. Who else would want to listen to me?" He barked as though saying he agreed with me. He was funny!

We now made our way out into the light again. I could see that my knees had been quite cut from the fall onto some jagged rocks and were now bleeding. But, I didn't have time to think about them for too long before I could see the fifth gate ahead of us. It was covered in many beautiful flowing green vines with pink and yellow flowers tugging them gently everywhere. But even through this I could see the gate's glittering gold bars.

As we moved closer to the gate, I noticed that this time, it had not been opened before we arrived. "Oh dear," I said out loud. "What do you think, Mr. Rickert? Is it time to rest?" He nodded in agreement; he was too tired to bark this time.

So, we sat down on a soft grassy spot, just in front of the last gate. "Well, Mr. Rickert, I don't know what the next belief is that I need to have to open this gate, but whatever it is, I want to thank you for being so nice to join me on this special journey to help my father get well." I said this kindly as he lay across my lap, trying to lick my knees.

Then, like magic, the fifth and final gate slowly creaked its way open! "Oh my," I gasped as I threw my hands to my mouth. "We did it again, Mr. Rickert! Somehow we opened the final gate."

I was so excited that I wildly looked around to discover what the final message had been. "Where is it?" I thought.

All of a sudden, I felt a lot of tingling in my heart area. I started to laugh. It was tickling me. I was really feeling joyful!

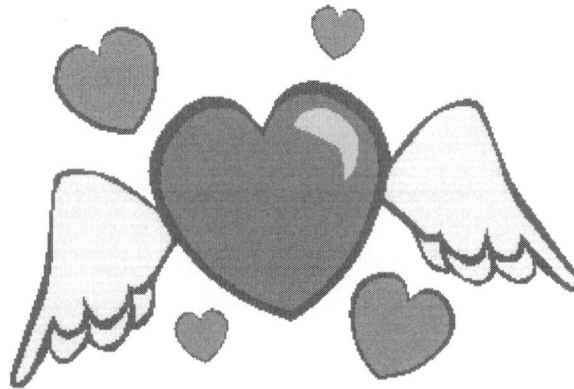

"Could it be, Mr. Rickert, that the last message is in my heart?" Mr. Rickert started twirling around in circles. How did he know that I too felt that I could spin around in circles?

I sat down again, breathless. I felt something poking at me, where I was sitting. I moved over slightly and saw a little piece of metal shining beneath the grass. I tapped it slightly and could now hear that it was a box of sorts.

I pulled away the grass and dirt around the metal, and was now certain that it was a beautiful little silver box with purple and red hearts painted around each side. I had trouble opening the box, from which dirt was now crumbling. But, at last I was able to peak inside it to find a heart shaped piece of metal that looked as though it were meant to be hung upon a necklace.

I could see that there was writing on this necklace. It said, **"Just for now, be kind."**

"Ah ha!" I yelled out to Mr. Rickert. "Just as I was being kind to you and you were being kind to me, the gate had opened! That wasn't so hard was it?" I laughed.

"Well, Mr. Rickert, let's go now and find whatever it is we need to help Father!"

We slowly walked through the gate and came upon a magical garden! It was so beautiful! I have never seen so many flowers! There were those shaped like birds and those shaped like musical instruments. Some looked like candy so tasty that I had to keep Mr. Rickert from eating them.

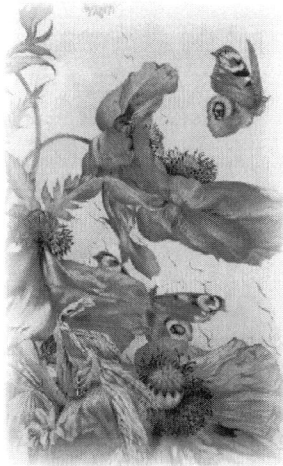

The ground was covered with a splendid green grass, so thick that my shoes disappeared into it as I walked. I was so involved in looking at everything around me that I almost forgot that I had to quickly find whatever it was that I needed to take to my father as soon as possible.

I now didn't know what to do. What was it I was looking for? Did I have to take a plant back to Father, or perhaps a piece of a flower? What about those wild vines hanging near the gate? Would I ever know what to take back for him? Would there be enough time left to help him?

"All right," I thought to myself. Maybe Mr. Rickert could sniff out what we needed. "Mr. Rickert," I yelled. "Come here, boy. I need your help!" Where was he? He wasn't answering.

"Mr. Rickert, where are you?" I yelled out again. "I need you! Come here boy!"

"Why wasn't he answering," I thought to myself. I hoped he wouldn't be gone for too long. I wanted to get back soon.

"Woof, woof, woof, squawk, squawk, squawk!" I heard repeated, over and over again from behind me. I turned around quickly to see orange and blue feathers flying in the air. Before I could catch myself, I was falling into a small little lake.

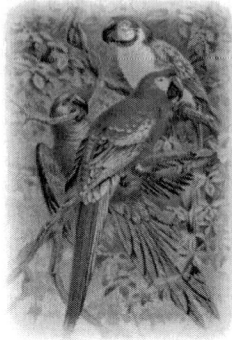

Then *SPLASH*! I fell with my whole body into Emerald coloured water, and then stood up quickly noting the knee height of the water. It was a mixture of both blue and green, and just glowed and glowed.

I stood there still and seemed to be waiting for the unwanted moment when slimy little silver fish would begin to swim between my legs. I was also afraid that little suckers would grasp onto a toe, like they often did at the lake near my home. But none came. In fact, there seemed to be no little critters in here at all.

My toes were squishing into a very soft surface, so I reached down to see what this was. When my hand again returned to the air, I was cradling sparkling golden sand.

"Very beautiful indeed," I thought to myself. "Not at all common to our lakes back home."

I chose then to leave the wonderful Emerald coloured lake, however warm and enjoyable, and continue my search for something that I could take back to help my father. I was on the grass again in a split second and sat down to let it soak up the water.

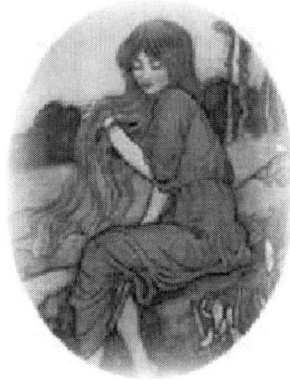

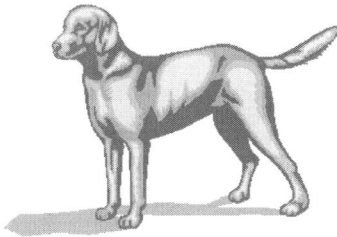

"How unusual," I said out loud, as I looked down at my knees that had been scraped. Then even louder I yelled, "They're almost gone…on my knees…the things…the scrapes, the cuts…oh my…they've gotten so much better!" I was in awe. I know I had scraped my knees up quite a bit when I fell. I had certainly felt a lot of pain. But, now the pain and most of the cuts were mostly gone. How amazing!

"This is it!" I yelled again. This excited yelling was getting to be a habit and it seemed to pull Mr. Rickert away from his playing with the birds. I had miraculously fallen into what I needed to take back to my father. It was contained within this Emerald lake. I was so thankful at that moment. Just when I thought I didn't know what to find, it found me. But, how would I take this water back to my father?

Mr. Rickert had now arrived at my feet and lay down. I could see that his nose had been cut during his play with the bird. So, I went and placed my hands on his back to soothe his pain. I could see that he was happy now and breathing very smoothly, not rushed like before.

His nose seemed to be getting better as well. It hadn't disappeared all at once, but it was slowly improving.

"Mr. Rickert," I hollered, startling him. "Do you think that it's now in my hands? That maybe somehow I carry whatever special thing it is that is in the water that helped me with my knees?" He woofed with enthusiasm!

Well, Mr. Rickert did tend to be right most often! I was going to trust that he meant *yes*!

"Okay, Mr. Rickert, let's go. We have to get back to Father!" Just then, I got up and started running for the gate. As I made my way through, I could hear Mr. Rickert trying to keep up, gasping for air.

I took it slower through the cave this time and finally made my way back to the winding path. It was here that I would always wonder what really happened. But, before I could even get excited about being closer to my father, I had fallen over the edge of the path and was tumbling through the trees towards the ground.

"Aaaahhhhh!" I was shouting as I felt Garin shaking me.

"Lolly. Lolly, wake up! Wake up. Are you okay? Sara, help me. She's screaming!" shouted Garin.

Then Sara began to shake me, as I slowly began to awaken. "My dear, what have you been dreaming about? You've given us all quite a fright. Except for Father, of course, who hasn't awoken yet."

"Father, Father!" I cried out, while everyone stood around looking baffled. "I'm back Father….I'm back!" I was now leaning over him and whispering into his ear. "I have carried the special Emerald water through my hands to help you. I don't know if it will work, but it helped me and whatever happens, I want you to know that I love you." Then, much like when I helped Mr. Rickert, I placed my hands on my father, taking a hold of both his hands.

I closed my eyes and imagined the bright water from the Emerald lake coming through my hands. They began to turn very hot, but I was not afraid at all. In fact, I felt quite full of love.

"Father!" Garin, Sara and I cried out at once, as we saw him begin to stir and heard him fumble with the words, "Don't let the dog in until you've dried his feet." We all laughed! We knew now that Father was going to be well! Mr. Rickert began to lick his face.

We all sat around him now, Garin and Sara each holding one of his large hands. Smiling down at him, I said I was sorry for taking such a long time to get back to help him. Sara and Garin both looked at each other wondering what I was talking about.

Sara said, "Lolly, what do you mean long time? We've all only been here for 10 minutes at best." Garin also agreed that that was true.

"Ten minutes?" I thought to myself. It took me a moment, and then I laughed. "Well here I am anyhow!" I said aloud.

"You are glowing!" Father tried to say loudly but was still very weak. "You are glowing!" he repeated. "It would seem that our travels together have given you something extra special that I can't quite put my finger on right now!"

I laughed again! "I have indeed found something extra special, Father! I have indeed!"

Hand Positions for Children 9 and under
When you begin, merely say, "I welcome the Reiki to flow."
When you complete, say, "Thank you for the Reiki. Its love and its protection!"

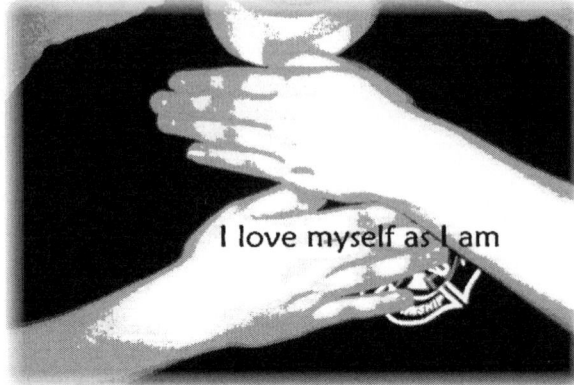

I love myself as I am

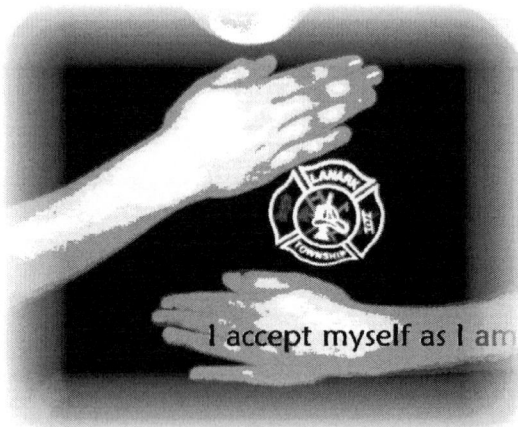

I love myself as I am

I accept myself as I am

A Gentle Reiki Hand Position to Help Another

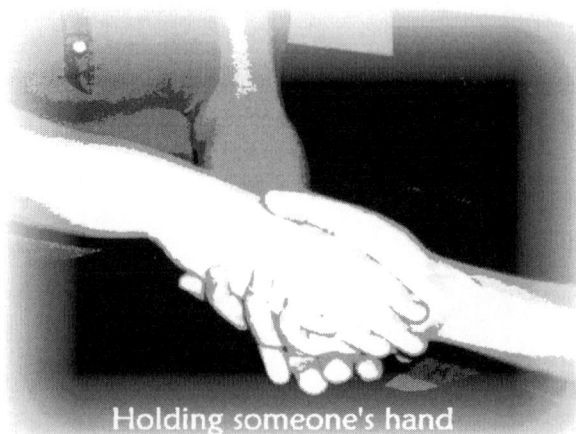

Holding someone's hand

Holding Someone's Hand

Mount Kurama and the Emerald Lake
10 years of age and over

If there was anything I wanted to know when I was a child, it was how my little white haired Great Aunt was able to help so many people release their aches and pains. She was grand, brilliant and terribly funny! She could also help you calm down after crying so hard that you felt your nose was going to blow off. She could look directly at you from across the room and suddenly you'd feel like someone was tugging at your ear or hugging you from behind.

She did all this with a twinkle in her eyes and laughter that was wonderfully hilarious! Aunt Lolly was a fun woman! She was so full of life and love that even my rough and tumble dog, Joshy, ran up to her and licked her old, soft and wrinkly face. Everyone wanted to be around her, she was abundantly happy and bubbly, so much so that everyone teasingly asked her what her secret was.

Each time, she would answer that she was born with a heart so overwhelmingly full of love that it poured over with nowhere else to go except out to everyone else. This she said, over and over, during the 13 long years that I knew her.

Then one year before she died, she pulled me aside and said that it was time to share the real story, the truth of her ability to help people by touching them with her hands or by sending them love. She said that she felt incredible peace and love inside. That was why others felt so greatly at peace in her company that they couldn't help but laugh and feel good. But, how she got to this great "feeling" place was such a special journey that only a young heart could truly understand its magic.

I was to promise only to tell the story of her experiences in the form of a myth. She said that a myth was a story that carried a message; some of it held facts and some of it was make-believe. This helped people to understand the messages within the story, in their own way and in their own time. It would encourage them to use their imaginations! It would allow more of their creative energy to flow in their lives. Then they could discover for themselves the secrets of the messages contained within the myth.

The key was then to use those messages to help themselves and other people live life with more love, which would help the world become more peaceful. She knew this was possible because she had lived it, and loved herself and others through it all. She was someone none of us could ever forget, and this is the fantastic mythical journey she shared with me.

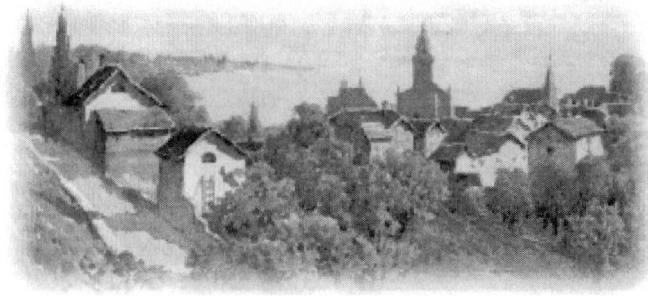

Lolly Shares Her Story

When I would look out the window of my tower room, I could see over the whole city of Crickmore. The Tower was as bright and magnificent as a lighthouse. It had been built a century before by a widowed woman, who, following the death of her husband, insisted upon a tower to overlook the city. She wanted to be able to find her children whenever they were out playing.

Mother and Father told us that they would never be as overly attentive as she had seemed to be and that when they wanted us home they would only ever have to yell out really loud. If we didn't respond and they had to send out our dog, Mr. Rickert, to find us, then we could really expect a talking to!

The windows of the tower glittered with the sun as it poured in everyday, in everyway.   I begged my mother not to put up drapes. I wanted to see and know everything that was going on around me as often as I was in my room, my sacred place. Instead, we hung huge swaths of cloth in upside-down rainbow shapes all along the walls, joining one to another, all connected, above and below my massive windows. There was bright red, yellow, orange, purple, blue, green and a really brilliant indigo.

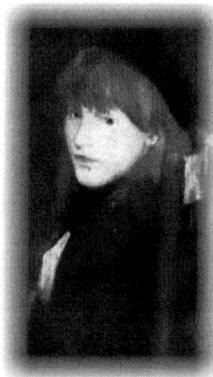

My little brother, Garin, called me Lolly, because he had trouble saying Lillian. He was only 3 at the time, so I forgave him. The new nickname stuck and I was from thereon Lolly to everyone, young and old. Even my father thought it was the funniest name. He would call me into the parlour by yelling out, "Ooohhhh Miss Lolly, Polly, Dolly. Would you please come down here for a moment? I'm wondering if you wouldn't mind joining me for a cup of tea!" He would laugh as he said my name, and then repeat it under his breath, with a chuckle, before he moved on to more serious matters.

One day he called my brother, now 8 years old, my older sister and me down to the parlour. He seemed more serious than usual, so I asked him what was wrong. He said that it was time for us to move. We had been in our home for 7 years; two years before my mother, Ada, had died, and now we were being told we were going to move. I couldn't believe my ears.

"But," he said more lively, slapping his hands on his bony knees, "we're going on a great big adventure to Japan!" Garin and I jumped up and down with joy. We had seen many pictures of Japan and had always wanted to go there. Our father had shown us the world with his atlas and then bought many picture books to let us see what each part of the world looked like. We were so excited that the room seemed to light up with our smiles. My older sister, Sara, however, just started to cry: probably another boyfriend problem. You know, at 16 she wasn't too smart. I mean who cares about boys anyway? They just take your stuff and make silly fart like noises with their mouth. Yuck!

Sara, or Teary Eyes as we liked to call her, was always crying over some lost boyfriend. If a boyfriend hadn't smiled at her properly that day she'd end up feeling so sad that she would spend at least an hour blowing her nose and wiping her eyes.

At 11 whole years of age, I was a lot more aware of these things! I knew that when you liked someone you certainly didn't run away if they didn't smile at you. Instead, you'd go up to them and ask them how they were. If they were having a bad day, you could understand why they didn't smile, and if they were just being grumpy and thoughtless, you could kick them in the shin and then tell them to grow up! Of course, you would have to have clear access to the out door and run like the wind, as my mother used to say.

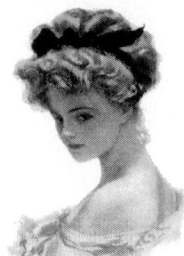

She was quite beautiful, my mother. She had the softest skin of anyone I had ever known, and she always smelled like daisies. She smiled like one too; she lit up so brightly. I missed her, but carried her picture with me always. I could feel her. She was never really far away.

My father was a doctor, and he said that there had been an awful earthquake in Tokyo, killing thousands of people and leaving many people hurt or ill. He was asked to go there by the head of the Crickmore Medical Association, and so we would all go. Father could never be away from us for too long. He always said he missed our quirky little habits that reminded him he was living in a circus. Then he'd tickle us until we couldn't bear it, leaving us like little puddles on the floor, too breathless to get up.

Our adventure was to begin in one week. Father had already spoken with his solicitors who would manage to rent our home while we were away. We would be gone for a year, maybe more. We were even to bring Mr. Rickert along.

There was so much to do. There were boxes piled on tops of tables and tables upside down on tops of boxes. Our home became a maze. Not even a mouse could find its way out without a map. I would call out to Garin and hear his cute squeaky little voice behind a box somewhere in the parlour, but it would take me 5 minutes darting in and out of boxes to find him. Finally, I would see him, clasp him in my arms and whirl him around, until I hit a box and we'd both tumble. He was still light enough for a little fun play.

It wasn't long before we were all ready to go. We said goodbye to our home and jumped into the new 1923 Packard my dad's friend, Mr. Sylvestrie, had just purchased. It was so long and shimmered in black. Mr. Sylvestrie said it was the newest Single Eight model, whatever that was supposed to mean. It was more comfortable than a saddle, but I didn't care much for motorcars; my horse, Gatherer, was far greater than any motorcar could ever be. He ran faster than the wind on some days. The motorcars also smelled poorly, not that Gatherer didn't leave smells behind him from time to time!

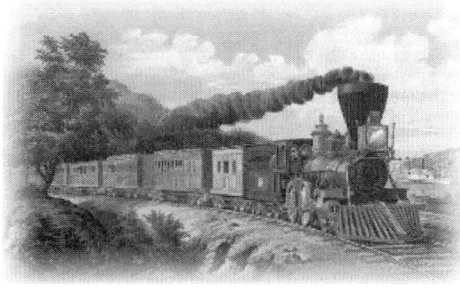

We travelled by motorcar for several hours, until we were sleepily guided onto a boat to France. We then journeyed through France on a train to Italy where we had to take another train and then another train, until we finally made it to the tip of the country. All the way down to the toe of the boot, as my father said. Italy looked like a boot on my father's atlas. Garin asked if that's why they made such good shoes there. He had apparently overheard some of Sara's friends talking about their favourite shoes.

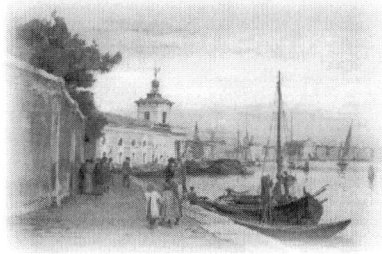

From Italy we travelled across the Mediterranean Sea to the Arab countries. Here we saw these huge animals called camels. They were taller than any horse I had ridden and I was allowed to climb upon one with Sara for a ride. Mr. Rickert jumped along enthusiastically beside us. He seemed excited to have made a new friend; the camel seemed to like him more that my horse, Gatherer, did.

The boy Azlam who guided the camel was my age and he thought he would scare us by running with the camel, which of course made Sara scream, but I wasn't afraid. I knew that if I fell into the sand I wouldn't hurt myself. I'd fallen from trees, so falling from a camel would be far less frightening.

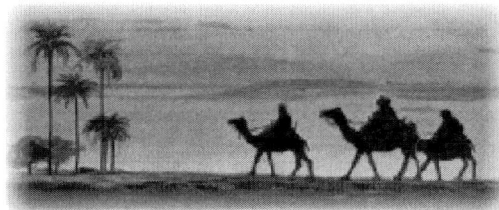

After two weeks of travel, my father finally said we deserved something of a holiday. Travelling might have been fun but it was also hard work at times! So, here we were in India, an amazing country. Father had a friend here named Sanjeev. Sanjeev's family consisted of one daughter, four boys and his wife, Lata, who had black hair that went all the way down to her waist. The robe she wore glistened in the light. It was so beautiful. One day she clothed me in one of her robes. She called it a "Sari." They were like dresses, but more flowing than I would have been allowed to wear back home. From shoulder to toe, I looked like a glimmering, walking rainbow. Every time I looked down, I'd laugh and laugh. I couldn't believe how much fun it was to wear a dress. I had never liked them before. But, here I was, feeling like a princess, unlike anyone I had known before.

Sanjeev, wearing his own creamy robe-like clothing, called a tunic, was also a doctor, who had trained with my father in our country.   But he came back to his homeland to work as a doctor. Then he got married and had a family with Lata. He spent many hours with my father, discussing the work he was involved in. He worked with a group of others that were trying to create a free homeland for Indians who were now under the rule of another country. The leader of this group was at that time in jail. I remember seeing a paper of sorts, called something like the Little India or the Young India. The leader had spent much time writing for it. Sanjeev had a copy in English and although I didn't understand all of the words and their meaning, I knew that this was important and that Sanjeev, his family and friends should also have complete freedom like me. I was going to be able to vote when I grew up. He couldn't even choose an Indian leader for his country. I told him that I would give him my vote if he wanted it, but he told me that he would become stronger if he could use his own voice. I wasn't sure what that meant, but he thanked me for my generous offer and we went off to share a dinner with everyone.

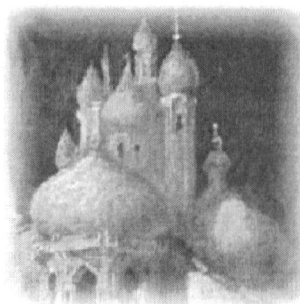

On the day we were to leave India, Lata's littlest child, her daughter Tara, ran up to me and wrapped her arms around me. She had the most soft and curly black hair I had ever felt. Her eyes were so round and beautiful that you could barely take your own eyes off of them. She looked up at me and said, "If you come back I'll build you a palace." We all laughed, while I squeezed her so hard that she squealed in delight! Everyone thought Tara didn't

meters from land or sea. Before we knew it, we were ready to go and were floating off towards Japan. Our destination was Tokyo and our pilot, named Chin, said that if we asked the Wind God to blow in the direction of Tokyo, which was North East of Shanghai, we would be there by the next morning.

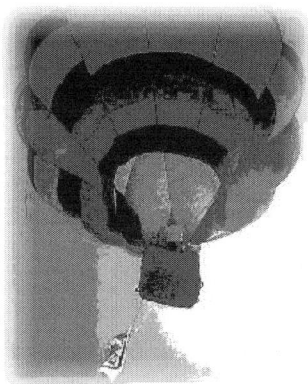

He had winked at us as we lifted off, each of us banging slightly against the sides of the basket. It didn't seem long before we were mid-way between China and Japan, above the East China Sea. Garin wanted to sit in the bottom and play a game of Snakes and Ladders, but I was too fascinated by what I was seeing to sit down. I kept moving from side to side of the basket, gazing out over the Sea. Fujio asked me what I was looking at because he believed that from every view, there was just Sea. We had long ago left sight of land.

I still felt the need to look out from every side of the basket. The experience had completely captured my excitement. I actually felt a different feeling each time I looked out from the many different sides of the basket. Most of the time we were close enough to the purple balloon that we could yell out to Sara and Father, and they would hear what we said. I could see from a distance that Sara was looking very pale, but Father no longer needed to have his arm around her. She seemed to be calming down and might soon become as adventurous as me… Or, on second thought, maybe not!

We slept through the night and by the time we awoke, Garin and I could see land. It was beautiful. Japan seemed to be a land that had seen thousands of years of amazing experience. At one point I could hear laughter and in the next I almost thought I had heard the sound of swords clashing with each other. Perhaps an echo of the earth's memory in the time of the Samurai warriors, my father had once told me about.

I had wandered off in my imagination of how Japan might have been in times not that long ago, when suddenly I saw my father's balloon begin to drop rather quickly. I heard Sara's screams and my heart began to beat so fast that I felt like I did during those times when I would run after my horse, Gatherer.

I yelled out to Chin, "Follow that balloon!" And down we went too, though not as quickly. Fujio had just a moment ago told us that we were now North of the city of Kyoto, still West of Tokyo. We could see a mountain ahead, which seemed to be buried in countless large cedar trees. It was here, at the foot of this mountain, that we were all to land.

I kept watch of the purple balloon, and was fearful that my family might not survive such a sudden fall from the skies. As they got closer to the base of the mountain, I could see that they were falling quickly. I heard a loud *WOOSH,* as they suddenly landed in a clear area of tall grasses. There was one final scream from Sara as the basket landed, fell over and seemed to flatten into the grasses.

I felt my heart stop beating for a moment and then I demanded Chin get us down immediately. Knowing my terror, he did not become angry with me for my lack of respect to him. He merely said that we would soon be with them, as the balloon was swiftly making its way near. I would later apologize.

By the time we landed we were still at least 150 metres or more from the other balloon. I jumped out quickly and ran with all my strength. Now was the time for me to put what my father called "my long giraffe legs" into motion.

As I arrived, practically crashing into the basket, I could hear nothing but a little whimper from Mr. Rickert. I yelled out and realized that I was standing in at least a couple feet of water. The basket had landed in water! What a relief! They had been given more of a cushy landing than I believed was possible from where they fell. I was finally able to look into the basket where I saw two of them rapidly breathing and Mr. Rickert licking his right back leg, which seemed to be motionless. It was certainly broken.

"Oh no. Mr. Rickert!" I said. "How can I help you?" I was reminded that there were actually three people in the basket. Sara seemed stunned but well, and the pilot was moving the hair from my father's eyes, attempting to look inside his eyes to see if he was still alive.

The pilot said he was breathing and before we knew it, Fujio, Garin and Chin were with us, each of them reaching to carry my father to a dryer place. Once we were all gathered together again, I overheard Garin ask Chin if any of us had done something wrong to make the wind God angry with us. Chin assured Garin that sometimes we cannot understand why things happen, but there was always a greater purpose to all that happened. We needed to trust that there were things that we could not yet know.

Garin seemed relieved to hear this answer and wandered over to Mr. Rickert, who was still nursing his wounded leg. I sat next to my father and asked him to wake up. But he didn't move. Sara and I began to cry. Her tears were from fear and mine were, of course, just because I was tired.

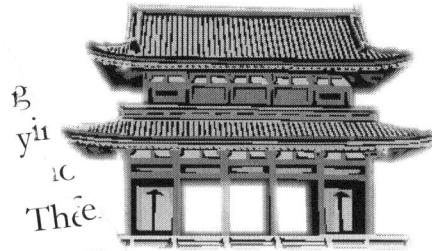

I then heard Fujio telling other pilot that this mountain before us was Mount Kurama. It was a sacred had a Buddhist temple mid-way up it. He said that there were several levels and that there were stories telling of healing powers, which could be gat fifth level of the mountain. I wondered what kind of levels a mountain could h

I was racking my brain over with the question of what I could now do. And my heart was aching to take action it so helpless! I felt so lost!

"Ah ha!" I said out loud. I away from the group and sat down next to a cedar tree that seemed to be on the out ge of the thousands of others beyond it. I was going to sit silent by and wait until I had an answer.

I seemed to be sitting for a lo time; over and over I would get lost in thought and stop listening to my breath. But the would try again and again to let my attention just happen without too much effort, until nally I was completely in silence. After a short time I found the way to my answer and knew what I was going to do.

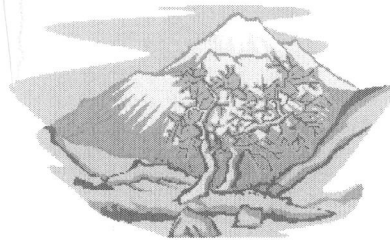

If there were ever a time to use my climbing skills, it was now. The sky was becoming red and a lot of time had seemed to pass. It was almost sunset. I knew that the sun always set in the West and could see it now beside the mountain. It rose each morning from the East to start a new day; and to create a new beginning. I would want to remember where the sun was so that I could find my way back to my family and our new friends if I got lost.

Here I was at the base of Mount Kurama. What a strong earth it must be to hold up such a large mountain. Perhaps the roots of all these trees also helped to hold it in place. I recalled the words of the seventh goddess; I would know what I had to do and have what I needed when I was called to my challenge. I also felt really peaceful in my decision and felt myself supported somehow, even with everybody focusing on my dad. So, just for now, I wasn't going to worry.

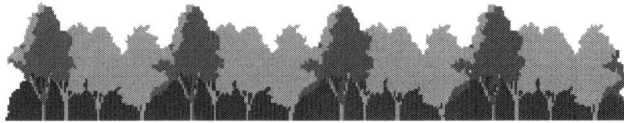

I also didn't want to worry everyone else, so I told only Garin what I was going to do. He trusted me, and he had no choice but to look up to me; I was taller than he was! I told him not to tell anyone until they saw that I was missing, and then he could just say that I had decided to go for a walk, but was marking my way back and would not be long. I had been taught to leave marks on trees in order to remember where I had been, so I could always get home.

In a matter of seconds, I had chosen which part of Mount Kurama I was going to climb. I was completely ready to go, and only needed something to mark my way, when I looked down and realized that there was something in my coat pocket. I reached in and recognized the reddish stone! It was the one given to me by the first goddess! How amazing! I could use this to mark my way.

I began to run, stopping briefly to mark the trees on my path. I could feel that I knew exactly where to go. I had no doubts, just faith in the journey. I was going to gather those healing powers at the fifth level of the mountain and help my dad wake up! I must now be on the first level. As I had been running now for some time, I could feel the brush of the cedars pushing me toward the mountain. They had heard that I was in need of help, and they had really listened and were helping me in the best way they could.

Now I could feel that I had to work harder to run. I realized that I had reached a different level of the mountain. It must be the second level. I was getting closer to what I wanted, but I knew that I just had to focus on where I was and not be distracted, because I might otherwise get really lost.

Then right out of the blue, there was a huge wall in front of me. I had reached a solid rock face. This wall of rock seemed only to have an edge on which I could again climb about 10 metres up. Now what was I going to do? I angrily threw my hands up in the air, but as they were falling, I thought to myself, "Just for the moment, I won't get angry." And I let my hands down more easily as they swiped the sides of my coat. Again I knew what I had to do. I wouldn't have noticed this at all if I hadn't let the anger go just for a moment.

The seed! The seed! Plant the seed and it will grow for you exactly what you need. Isn't that what the second goddess had said? It was all coming back to me now! I believe! I believe! I can do this. I waited for another moment. Then I gently pulled the seed from my other coat pocket. I had never actually looked closely at the seed before now.

It glowed a bright orange and was surrounded in a golden light. I looked down upon it as I cradled it in my hands. I drew it closer to my body, and as I did, it became even brighter. Finally it was right next to my coat, in my hands, and just below my belly button. The tremors were very sudden as the seed quickly expanded to the size of a football and its light entered me as I continued to shake.

This was more troubling an experience than I had yet had on our travels. The seed was gone; I was shaking and my father was hurt at the bottom of a mountain in Japan. I wished I were home in my old bed, with its four posters and swaying drapes, hanging from ceiling to post. It was my own little safe tent and I longed to swing again on the rails between the bedposts.

I was tired and so kneeled down to rest. I felt rumblings occurring where the light of the seed had entered me. I was not at all sure whether it was me who was rumbling or whether there was something inside me growing. I stood up in discomfort and gathered some soil in my hands as I did so. The soil began to grow into something that looked like a brick and became so heavy that I almost fell over with it as it tumbled to the ground. I felt lightness then.

The brick became larger and larger and then another brick was being created on top of that one, and then another and then another. Soon I recognized the creation as a set of stairs, becoming as tall as the rock face, and capable of taking me to the next level of the mountain. As I walked these steps I knew that my thoughts had been heard.

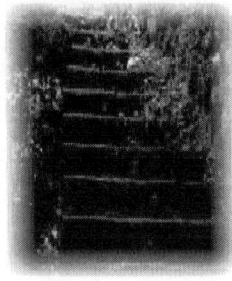

What a sense of relief reaching that last step! I had reached a new level, with a sense of joy. The seed had been planted inside me and my will to take that next step had allowed that seed to grow into something absolutely perfect for my climb of Mount Kurama.

I looked before me and saw only trees. The path was so unclear and yet I was in awe. I had never before seen such beautiful green trees. Their branches seemed to be reaching out to me, as though trying to embrace me. There were two in particular just to my right that seemed to call out to me and beckon me. I was now learning to trust myself more and to know that I was being guided to where I could most help my father. With this in mind it was easy to continue walking towards the trees, feeling gently guided to do so.

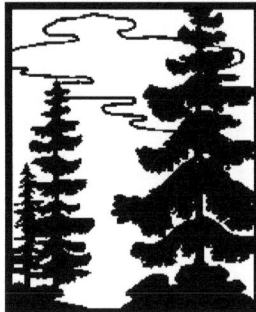

Standing before these two trees, I soon felt myself pulled between them. They had shown me the direction I needed to take. I knew that I would be shown the direction I needed to take from time to time, but that in this moment the hard work ahead was up to me.

I trudged along, comforted by the surrounding cedar trees. They blocked out most of the sun, but there was enough light to see a path ahead that seemed to have been trodden by others before me. I could see a clearing and in that place I could see a temple, much like the one I had seen in China. I thought that maybe I would find someone there to help me get to the fifth level of the mountain, but just as I breathed a sigh of relief, I heard the movement of branches and saw two trees immediately to my left that were calling me towards them.

"Oh my! This wasn't going to be easy," I said to myself. But, I was still willing to work hard, so I followed their guidance.   It seemed that the more I listened and allowed myself to accept that the trees were guiding me, the more that this once frightening journey was beginning to flow more comfortably. Once I had made the choice to work hard and pay attention, suddenly everything became easier.

Someday I was going to have to tell this story. It felt so significant; I knew it could change people's lives. I couldn't imagine who would believe it, but that was just fine. I would have fun telling it!

As I walked through the branches of the cedars, I again felt that I was being embraced and comforted. This time there was no path that had been walked on. In fact, I felt as though I was wading through a couple of feet of long ago fallen cedar needles that seemed to be turning yellow. There were still birds, with their twittering and wings flapping, and there were little critters, sometimes running between the trees, which reminded me of the small forest behind our home in Crickmore.

Just as I let my mind wander, I hit another wall of rock! "Oh, no. Oh, no!" I yelled to myself. Why did the trees guide me here? Having stopped paying attention for a moment, I seemed to have lost my way. So, I turned around to see if the trees had a new direction for me, but they didn't. Then I heard a noise to my right, as a large bird shook the branches of a tree. And there beneath the bird were the branches of two trees guiding me in their direction.

I brushed up against many branches as I passed between these two trees; they seemed closer than the ones I had previously passed by. Then, there again was another wall! This time I was so angry. I yelled out very loudly, "Father, why did you bring us on this outrageous journey!"

Catching my anger, I said, "Oh Father, I am sorry for being angry. I know you have done your best and want us all to be safe and happy. I understand why you have brought us all with you and in this moment, I will try to be kind."

And there it was. I noticed its dark ridges, and its clear markings. It was a map! A very large map, engraved onto the rock before me, which looked like it had been there for centuries. There were animals drawn next to it, a beautiful bird in the direction of North, a large elephant in the direction of South, a galloping horse to the West and a kneeling Llama to the East.

The map marked very clearly the levels of the mountain. There seemed to be seven. But I only needed to get to the fifth. Thankfully. I wouldn't have to climb too much further by the look of the map. The fifth level was clearly marked and it seemed that without even knowing it, I had entered the fourth level as I had walked into the wall. Odd really, finding yourself at a new level when hitting a wall.

On the map, there was an arrow that seemed to point into the wall. "Into the wall?" I questioned. "Oh my! That's it!" I said quite loudly outside myself. I could now see that somehow the fourth level was inside the mountain, because the wall before me seemed to go up and up forever. I had to find the entrance. The map seemed to show that just to the East, was a large opening in the mountain.

I brushed my way quickly through all of the branches in the way and then at once landed directly in front of the opening. I ran in, excited about having found this opening by being able to correctly read the map. The inside wasn't as dark as I had thought it would be. For some reason it seemed lit by a fuzzy green light. There were cobwebs in several places, and many different types of rock piles. Like little sculptures, all throughout this cavern. It wasn't even damp or cold, as I would have thought a cavern in a mountain would be. In fact, I felt warm and completely safe. As I walked forward, I could see that there was a ledge in one of the walls, which seemed to have countless candles on it. I wondered if this had been used as a type of shrine; a place where people could thank or pray to their God, and feel that he or she was listening.

It felt like that loving moment in Tibet during my daydream when my mother had hugged me. Perhaps I was experiencing this now because I was very much into the heart of the mountain and again being mothered by its opening to me. I again knew that she was near, because I could feel my heart expanding.

I cried out, "Hello, Mother. I love you!" I felt lighter and freer. I felt this way sometimes too, when I would ride Gatherer and we would be galloping together through one of the county fields. We were both one, riding with the force of everything we had to give. It was my way of being kind to myself while having incredible fun!

I heard the echo of my voice. Ahead of me I could see at least four entrances to a deeper part of the mountain. But there was only one entryway that seemed to reverberate with the echo of my voice, so that was the one I chose to enter.

"Thank you, Mother, for showing me the way!" I yelled out with joy. This cavern was terribly dark, but I could see more of the green light at the end of the passage. I walked forward much slower than my usual pace. I was afraid of stepping into another wall. I wasn't sure if it was easier to walk into a wall or walk into the dark. Perhaps they were the same.

All at once I tripped and skinned my right knee. It really hurt! I was feeling rather silly, although nobody else was there to see this happen. I was getting cranky with myself. But I knew my father would want me to be kind to myself. After all, this was no ordinary adventure and I was trying my best.

Just as I said this to myself, I could see the green light ahead of me become brighter and light up this new cavern much more than it had before. Finally, nearer to my goal!

"Hold on Father, I'm going to get you what you need! I'll be there soon!" I said to myself.

Now I was running again, thinking about the many times when I was younger that Mr. Rickert would come up and lick my face when I had fallen. I was so close to the end of the tunnel and then suddenly…………………………..I was there!

Wow! Before me was a lush garden, so full of plants with magnificently coloured flowers: all the colours of the rainbow, and even some I don't think I'd ever seen before. Some of them were as large and round as my head. The ground was covered with a luscious green grass, so thick that my shoes disappeared into it as I walked. I was so involved in looking at everything around me that I almost forgot that I had to quickly find the healing source so that I could get it to my father as soon as possible.

I didn't know what to do. What was it that I was looking for? Did I have to take a plant back to Father, or perhaps a piece of a flower? What about those wild vines hanging along the rock faces surrounding this garden? Would I ever know what to take back for him?

For some reason, I knew now that I must use the dream in Tibet as my guide. I was here on the fifth level of the mountain and recalled the words of the fifth goddess. "From your voice will come much power. Be unafraid to use it wisely and lovingly."

All right, I thought to myself. If I am to use my voice, is there something special that I should say or yell, or sing! "That's it," I yelled out. "I will sing again!"

And as before, I was suddenly able to use my voice as though calling out to the world around me to answer my call for help, and I sang out the note, "SOoooooooooooooo!"

It was brilliant. The tone was superb! I could see the flowers around me shaking like the chandelier would have, and the vines even began to tremble. Then as the note still reverberated, the vines behind the greatest bunch of bluish flowers all fell to the ground. Set back behind the vines was a little valley, tucked inside the mountain, and in the middle of this valley, was a brilliant little lake. It was the intense green of emeralds, like the five emeralds on the ring my mother used to wear. She said that each emerald was for the priceless beauty of each member of our little family.

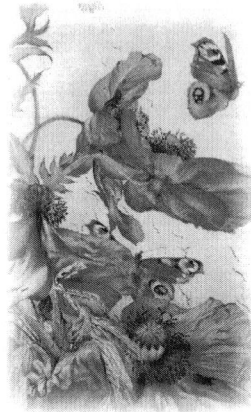

I walked hesitantly towards the lake that was drawing me to it with a vibrant ray of light. Except for the ray, the lake was completely still. There was no one else around. I was surprised because it seemed like a paradise, which could make even the grumpiest person begin to stir with joy.

I wasn't long beside the Emerald Lake when I heard what sounded like large birds squawking loudly behind me. As I turned around to look, I lost my footing and became completely unbalanced. I tried helplessly; flailing my arms in the air, to grasp what wasn't there to reach.

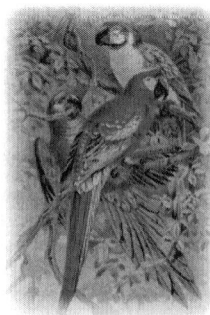

Then *SPLASH*! I fell full body into the Emerald water, and stood up quickly noting the knee height of the water. I seemed to be waiting for the unwanted moment when slimy little fish would begin to swim between my legs. I was also afraid that the little suckers would grasp onto a toe, like they often did at the lake near my home. But none came. In fact there seemed to be no little critters in here at all.

My toes were squishing into a very soft surface, so I reached down to see what this was. When my hand returned to the air, I was cradling sparkling, golden sand.

"Very beautiful indeed," I thought to myself. "Definitely uncommon to our lakes back home."

I decided to leave the wonderful Emerald Lake, however inviting, and continue my search for the healing power I needed to help my father. I was on the edge of the lake again in a split second and sat down to let the rocks and grasses capture the water from my dress and hair.

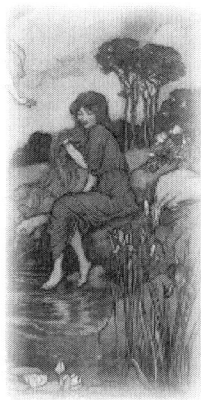

"How unusual," I said out loud, as I looked down at my knee that had been injured. Then even louder I yelled, "It's almost gone…my knee…the thing…the scrape, the cut…oh my…it's almost gone!" I was in awe. I know I had scraped my knee quite a bit when I fell. I had certainly felt a lot of pain. But now the pain and the cut were both so much better. How amazing!

"This is it!" I shouted again. This excited yelling was getting to be a habit. I had miraculously fallen into the healing power. It was contained within the Emerald Lake. I was so grateful in this moment. Just when I thought I didn't know what to do, everything I needed had arisen. Isn't that what the seventh goddess had said? I seemed to have been reminded of this a lot today.

I looked up and could see that there were at least two other levels to this Mount Kurama. I would definitely want to come back one day to explore them, but today, most importantly I had to get back to help my father with this healing power.

As I looked up to a place that would most likely have been the sixth level of the mountain, I remembered that the sixth goddess had told me that I was capable of not only using all of my five senses all the time, but that I had another sense. I finally figured out that this sixth sense was one that would allow me to know things without having been taught them.

I was reminded of those moments when I would ask my mother how she knew that it would rain that night, or how she knew that Sara would be late from school that day. I can remember her telling me several times, as she rested on the sofa that she just had a "GUT" feeling. I now knew what she meant.

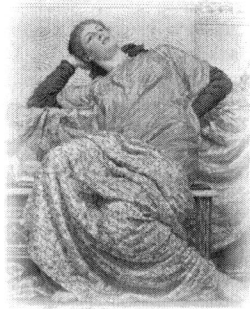

I suddenly knew that having been in the Emerald Lake, I now carried the healing power through me. I could use my hands, or even my thoughts to offer healing power. It could be offered only with love though and would always do what it was supposed to do, even if I didn't know what was really going on inside someone when I tried to help him or her. It would be one of those times of being quiet, which my father so enjoyed.

"All right!" I said quite clearly. "I am ready to go! Thank you!" I yelled out gratefully, to whatever it was that had shown me the way. I would never forget this experience, that was for sure. I now needed to find my way down from the mountain. If it was as challenging and as long as the journey up, I would most certainly not get back to Father before dark.

The words, "Be where you are!" at once loudly entered my head. "That's odd," I thought to myself. Was this one of those sixth sense moments again?

Suddenly, I felt the earth shaking beneath me and directly before me there was a gaping hole that had opened into the earth. I looked down into it and it seemed to be well-lit with a glowing white light. There appeared to be a slide of sorts inside. "A slide! How fun!" I thought.

"Well, I guess I've found my way home!" I joyfully stated. "Here I go!" I jumped onto the slide quickly and seemed to be barreling down at a very fast pace. Along the sides of the walls, there were images of my family that were always changing. I had seen slide shows like this in the big city with my father when we went in for medical supplies. But, this was far more exciting than the black and white images I had seen before. This was full colour! Wow!

Then, all at once "Bang!" I was back, swiftly seated beside a cedar tree near my father's unmoving body. It was like I had blinked from one moment to the next, and found myself exactly where I had started, but feeling different!

"Father. Father!" I cried out, while everyone stood around looking baffled. "I'm back Father....I'm back!" I was now leaning over him and whispering into his ear. "I have carried the healing power to help you. I don't know if it will work, but it helped me and whatever happens, I want you to know that I love you." Then I had a gut feeling that I should place my hands on either of the temples on his head.

I closed my eyes and imagined the ray from the Emerald Lake, a stunning shiny green, coming in through the top of my head, swirling around in my heart and then passing down into my arms and hands. They began to vibrate and became very hot and all the while, I felt such a sense of peace. I was not afraid at all. In fact, I felt quite full of love.

"Father!" Garin, Sara and I cried out at once, as we saw him begin to stir and heard him fumble with the words, "Don't let the dog in until you've dried his feet." We all laughed! Father was definitely going to be well! Mr. Rickert began to lick his face.

We all sat around him now, Garin and Sara each holding one of his large hands, while I sat to one side of his head with my hand on top of it. Smiling down at him, I apologized for taking such a long time to get back. Sara and Garin both looked at each other confused.

Sara said, "Lolly, what do you mean long time? We've only been here for 10 minutes at best." Garin nodded in agreement.

"Ten minutes!" I thought to myself. It took me a moment, and then I laughed. "Of course!" It would only take but one moment to have the experience of a lifetime. "Well, here I am anyhow!"

"And glowing!" Father tried to say loudly but was still very weak. "You are absolutely glowing! It would seem that our whole journey together has given you something extra special that I can't quite put my finger on right now!"

I laughed again, knowing that I was indeed forever changed. There was no turning back now. I again had one of those gut feelings that told me I was going to be sharing the lessons I had learned in my daydream in Tibet and during my journey up Mount Kurama.

It didn't matter where we went next, as long as we were together. I knew that whatever was to come for us was going to be really magnificent!

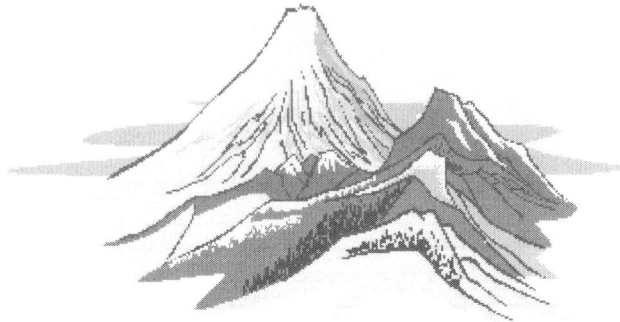

Later, around a fire, Fujio stated that he had been raised to believe that Mount Kurama had been a volcano that had come up from the sea. His grandmother had told him that every part of that mountain was connected to everything else in the world, through the sea where it had been created. As he went on intensely about the many levels of Mount Kurama, I thought to myself smiling largely, inside and out, "I know Fujio! I know!"

Reiki Hand Positions and Affirmations

When you begin, simply say, "I welcome the Reiki to flow."
When you complete, say, "Thank you for the Reiki. Its love and its protection."

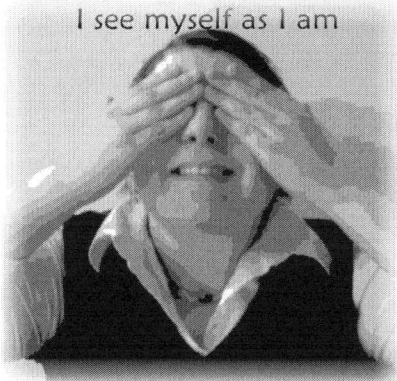

I see myself as I am

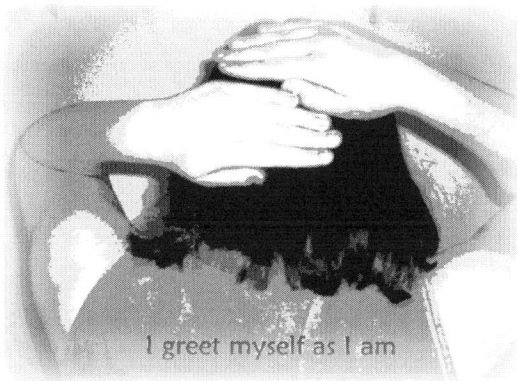

I greet myself as I am

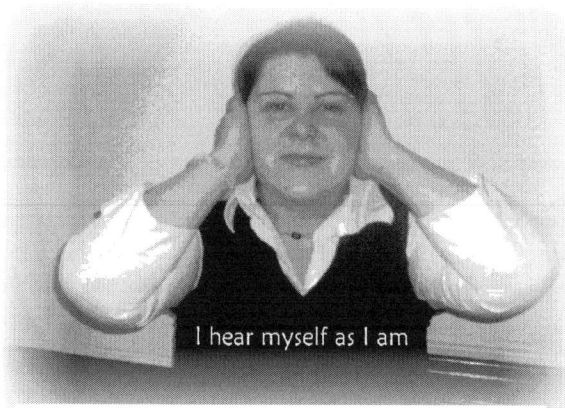

I hear myself as I am

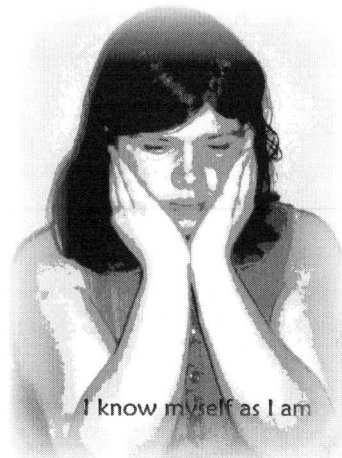

I know myself as I am

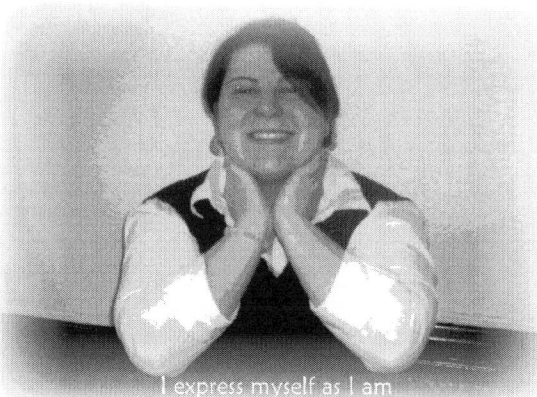

I express myself as I am

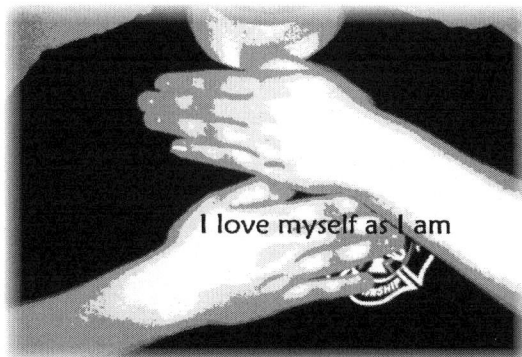

I love myself as I am

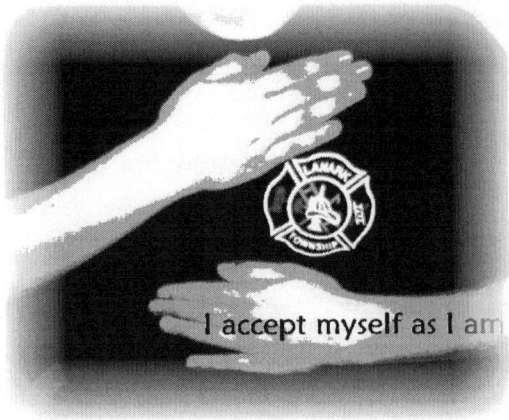

I accept myself as I am

Three Gentle Reiki Hand Positions to Help Others

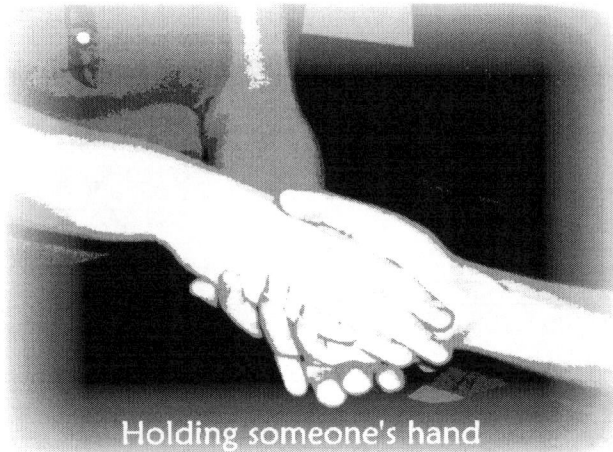

Holding Someone's Hand

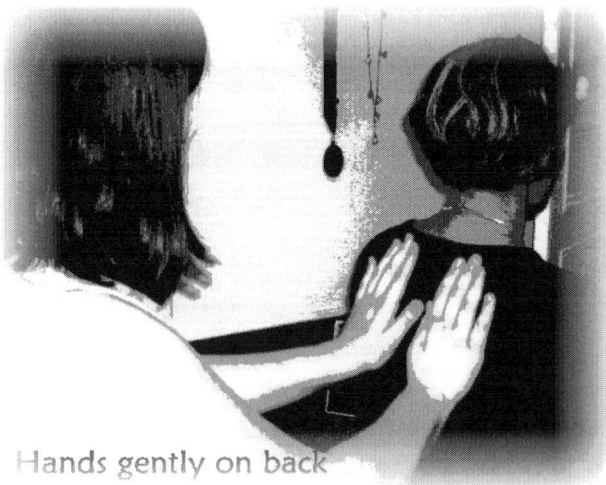

Hands gently on back

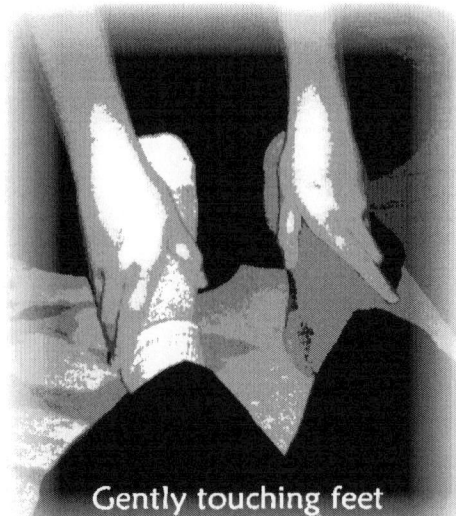

Gently touching feet

Insights

This section is to assist the parent, Reiki teacher and educator in understanding the different insights that have been placed within the stories for the young reader. They are similar for both stories, but there are significantly more within the longer story. Only the more obvious lessons/insights are noted here. There are many smaller statements that could be understood in other ways. These have been kept simple, and are only a cursory view of greater lessons stemming from the initial insight.

The Tower Room

Lolly has decorated her room with cloth that looks much like rainbows and has also been created from the colours of the chakras (swirling energy vortexes).

The Vote in India

Lolly learned that the value of having a vote was the opportunity for an individual to use his/her own voice and be heard. The writer of the newspaper that Lolly looks at is actually Gandhi, who was in prison at that time.

Foresight in India

As a little girl, Tara promised to build Lolly a palace if she came back. It turned out that she ended up as an architect who was asked to help a family friend build a palace. Sometimes people are so surrendered/open to the world around them that they can anticipate things to come without knowing how this arises.

Chakra Colours

Throughout the story, the colours of the chakras are used. There are seven main Chakras. The colours are found within the cloth hung in Lolly's bedroom, the dresses of the Goddesses and on the levels of the mountain. The sixth and seventh levels are not represented with a colour in the longer story.

1st Chakra- Red- the Root- representing foundation and solidity
2nd Chakra- Orange- the Sacral Chakra – representing creativity
3rd Chakra- Yellow- the Solar Plexus – representing the emotions and/or the mind (philosophies vary here)

4th Chakra- Green- the Heart Chakra – representing the centre of our love/feelings
5th Chakra- Blue- the Throat Chakra- representing our expression and its many powers
6th Chakra- Indigo- the Third Eye- representing our inner seeing and sixth sense/intuition
7th Chakra- White/Purple- the Crown Chakra- representing our divine connection

First Goddess

She represents the awareness of foundation, and of offering support, strength and courage. She shows Lolly that she is able, with this foundation in place, to reach beyond what she would otherwise believe to be true in her life. She is beginning her journey and is shown that she will be supported in this. The symbol of a small rock is used.

"It is from this rock that you will have the gift of being supported and the strength and courage to reach beyond what you think you know to be true."

Second Goddess

She represents Lolly's potential for creativity and notes the profound potential through love. She supports positive self-belief.

"In each moment, I was blossoming like this seed would also bloom one day. I was allowed to place this seed in my other pocket and she told me that when I was ready to plant it, it would grow quickly. I was supposed to plant it with love and it would then grow for me whatever I needed the most in that moment. Even if I wasn't really sure what it was I needed, I just had to believe."

Third Goddess

She represents the perfection of the mental/emotional part of the self when in balance. The pages are blank and the water flows easily without obstacle. This represents how easily our thoughts and emotions can flow when we are in a state of balance. The blank pages await Lolly's flow, so that she can write her experience and share it with others, so that they too might receive such flow.

"And what about the book? Why are the pages blank?" I retorted.

"One day all that you think and feel will flow as easily as this water," she repeated. And then she was gone.

Fourth Goddess

She represents the heart, which is the area where the soul is said to reside. Within this place is our perfection. From here we can feel and know that we are not alone, and we are living in connection and interdependence with all that is. In the expansion of our heart we can feel that connection even more profoundly and feel that we are receiving the love or the hug of the universe.

"Within your heart is the essence of everything -- even me. I am always with you. You need never fear being alone." She then asked me to close my eyes and I felt the area of my own heart expanding and becoming bright. In that moment, I felt as though I were being hugged."

Fifth Goddess

She represents the expression of the self and the centre of our personal power. She asks Lolly to know that her voice has power. When she uses it appropriately, she can effectively clear the way before her.

"From your voice will come much power. Be unafraid to use it wisely and lovingly."

"I was glad to sing so beautifully. Did my voice really have power?"

Sixth Goddess

She represents the capacity for seeing what would appear to be beyond our capacity to see. The inner seeing is available to each of us. Lolly was able to see that she had a sixth sense (intuition) and could use it for her highest good.

All of my senses were fully present and I then heard a voice that seemed to be coming from the Goddess before me, although she wasn't moving her mouth. She said, "You can smell, sense, feel, see, hear, and then realize all you need to, when you ask." I counted the senses she stated and then realized that there were six of them and not just the five senses I had been taught in school.

Seventh Goddess

She represents the connection to the whole. She is all knowing and all seeing from that greater vantage point. She further represents the support that this connection provides. She is wise and omniscient, and assists Lolly in knowing that everything from the whole (universal consciousness) is available to her in each moment.

"If you asked me to carry you over and over, I would, and when you are ready to know the truth, you will find me."

"As for now, you will very soon be asked to use some of the experiences you have gathered here today. You will be called to a great challenge. Finally...remember that you have all that you need, and you are all you need to be in each moment"

Borders between Tibet and China

Garin notes that there doesn't seem to be a change in the landscape as they enter China. He can't believe that they are leaving Tibet and entering another country. His father points out that borders are created in the minds of people. If we want to believe that there is a border, there will be; it is a state of mind.

Stillness/Silence

When Lolly and Garin get lost, she notices that when she is fully still and focused only on her breath, she can really hear what it is she needs to know to help the two of them. She heard the bell and was able to quickly remember that there had been a bell in front of the Buddhist Temple where her father and Sara were.

Climbing Mount Kurama and Passing through the Gates and Levels of the Mountain

Climbing Mount Kurama is like climbing the numerous mountains that we are each asked to climb in our lives. The many levels and gates of the mountain relate to the chakras and the experiences of the different initiations we are asked to face in our lifetime. As we pass through each level or gate, we release old perceptions and open to new insights that assist us in remembering our most authentic self, essentially, the perfection within. Lolly is remembering what is already within her. She is graduating from one level to another and is, interestingly, moving forward while sitting still. Lolly is climbing an internal mountain, which is often more difficult than any other. She is opening to her deepest truth, leading to a permanent shift in her consciousness.

First Mountain Level

This level is also associated with the message of the first Goddess. It represents the foundation upon which the other levels of the Mountain can rest. The gift of the stone was to let Lolly know that she would always be supported. The foundation is always the first step of a significant journey.

First Mountain Gate

This gate is associated with the Reiki principle which states, "Just for today I will not worry." Here Lolly is taught that when believing she need not worry, what would seem to be a challenge can simply pass away, or in this case, "open" so she can pass through.

Second Mountain Level

This level is associated with the message of the second Goddess.
It represents the level of creation. The seed is the metaphor for creation. From here, Lolly was able to inspire a set of stairs, coming from the direct creative part of her self. A part which each of us has within.

Second Mountain Gate

This gate is associated with the Reiki principle which states, "Just for today I will not anger." Here Lolly is taught that when believing she need not anger, the way through is clearer and she can get to where she needs to be more easily without attaching to any one moment of discomfort so that it is continued or extended further.

Third Mountain Level

This level is associated with the message of the third Goddess. It represents the emotional/mental level. At this level, Lolly was paying attention, listening and watching for the cues, or signs, that would guide her further. With this time of quiet attention she was more able to allow her mental/emotional self to come into balance. Therefore, the metaphor of the flowing water refers to her life being made easier because experiences, thoughts and feelings more gently flow through.

Third Mountain Gate

This gate is associated with the Reiki principle which states, "Just for today I will show gratitude." Here Lolly is taught that thankfulness is another important aspect to clearing the way on her path. Gratitude softens our hearts.

Fourth Mountain Level

This level is associated with the message of the fourth Goddess. This represents the heart/feeling level. Lolly is facing another wall and cannot see where she needs to go. Turning, she sees a Buddhist Temple and mistakenly believes that this is her intended destination. But instead she is guided to a path less travelled; a path that is just for her. She is shown how some journeys, although unclear in their direction, can still lead one to his/her destination. On her own path she finds further guidance and support through the images on a map.

It is here that Lolly remembers her mom again and through their loving connection is assisted by further guidance. Lolly is again reminded that she is never alone, but is always supported and guided. The heart is the centre of our connection to that place within us that is ever aware and loving.

Fourth Mountain Gate

This gate is associated with the Reiki principle which states, "Just for today I will work hard." Here Lolly is taught that hard work pays off. Not only did she believe this already, but also it is fully supported by the opening of the gate.

Fifth Mountain Level

This level is associated with the message of the fifth Goddess. This represents the centre of our expression, and its creative and powerful nature. With the use of her voice, Lolly can see the power even one note can have in creating change.

Fifth Mountain Gate

This gate is associated with the Reiki principle which states, "Just for today I will be kind." Here Lolly is taught that kindness is an additionally important aspect of making her life easier and more pleasing.

Compassion/Understanding

Lolly has taken her adventure up Mount Kurama as a way of helping her father. Her journey is one of first exhibiting and then cultivating compassion and respect. She is being called to attend to a purpose beyond her own self-need. She is showing her capacity for caring and understanding.

Sea of Life

Mount Kurama rose from the sea as a volcano. Everything is created out of one great "sea" of energy.

The Illusion

Lolly believed that she had been on an extended journey, only to discover that the whole family has only been there for 10 minutes. Lolly seems to easily have understood that everything was occurring in the one moment. With this in mind, she has touched upon the illusion that we all live in. Not only is everything connected through the sea of energy we are all a part of, and not separate from, but also we only need one moment in time to have a full experience.

Sharing

Through her experience Lolly is showing the importance of sharing what she has been given, and offering it for the highest good of another.

Self-Assurance/Self-Acceptance

Lolly is a very adventurous and self-reliant young girl. She has no problem taking charge of a situation and effecting change. She seems very comfortable with her self and shows how important it is to pursue one's honourable intentions.

Reiki Principles

At each level or gate of the Mountain, there is a Reiki principle that is stated in some way. By living with these principles, it is believed that one can live a quality, healthy and honourable life. The principles are sometimes written in different ways, i.e. the principle of being kind has been noted as, "Honour my teachers, parents and elders."

The principles are made more evident in the shorter story. They are most subtle and shared in a different order in the longer story. The order of the principles is not important as in the order of chakras.

The Five Reiki Principles as stated in the story for children 9 years and under

Just for today I will not worry. (1st Gate)
Just for today I will not anger. (2nd Gate)
Just for today I will work hard. (4th Gate)
Just for today I will be kind. (5th Gate)
Just for today I will show gratitude. (3rd Gate)

The Five Reiki Principles as stated in the story for children 10 years and over

Just for today I will not worry. (1st Level)
Just for today I will not anger. (2nd Level)
Just for today I will work hard. (3rd Level)
Just for today I will be kind. (4th Level)
Just for today I will show gratitude. (5th Level)

*(Please note that the principles arise at different times in the stories for different age groups)

Questions to Ask the Children for Reinforcement

These questions will help the children remember the story as well as the many lessons within. Please feel free to ask as many or few as you feel can be accommodated in the time you share with your child/student. These are just guides for your time together.

Story for those 9 years of age and under

- Do you remember what colours were in the cloth that Lolly hung up in her room?
- What kind of room was that?
- What could she see from her room?
- What was the message that Lolly had to believe to get through the first gate?
- What was the message that Lolly had to believe to get through the second gate?
- What was the message that Lolly had to believe to get through the third gate?
- What was the message that Lolly had to believe to get through the fourth gate?
- What happened to Lolly in the cave?
- What was the message that Lolly had to believe to get through the fifth gate?
- What did Lolly discover the Emerald water could do?
- How did she know that she could now take back the special quality of the Emerald water to her father?
- What did Lolly finally do to help her father?
- Where did she place her hands?
- Was this just a dream for Lolly?
- Do you believe all of the messages that Lolly believes?
- What were those messages?
- Can you use the special Emerald water to help yourself or others like Lolly did?

Story for those 10 years of age and older

- Do you remember what colours were in the cloth that Lolly hung up in her room?
- What kind of room was that again?
- What could she see from her room?
- Through which countries did she take a train?
- What kind of animal did she ride in the beginning of her Eastern Journey?
- What was it that Sanjeev (pronounced sunjeev) could not do in his country?
- When she was in India, what did the little girl Tara want to build for Lolly?

- Do you think that Tara somehow knew that someday she would end up building a palace?
- What or who is the Dalai Lama?
- How is the Dalai Lama found by the Monks?
- What country is he from?
- How many Goddesses visited Lolly?
- What did the first Goddess give Lolly?
- What did the second Goddess give Lolly?
- What do you think the Goddesses were trying to teach Lolly?
- What was the book for?
- What did the fourth Goddess have over her heart?
- What did Lolly see?
- Do you think Lolly would ever again feel alone after what she learned from the 4th Goddess?
- What did the fifth Goddess teach Lolly?
- What does it mean to use your voice?
- How many senses do you have? To taste etc….
- What was the sixth sense that Lolly had not been taught in school?
- What is the main message of the seventh Goddess?
- Do you know what the seventh Goddess meant when she told Lolly that she had all she needed and was all she needed to be in each moment?
- Why was Garin surprised as he entered China with his family?
- Do you believe it to be true that only men/women create borders between countries in their minds?   Was the earth created with borders? Are borders that important?
- While in China, Lolly and Garin got lost. How did they find their way back to their father and sister?
- What did being still or silent allow Lolly to do?
- What type of transportation did Lolly and her family use to get to Japan?
- What is the name of the Mountain that their balloons landed near?
- Where did Fujio say the healing energy could be found?
- How many levels are there on the mountain?
- Why do you think there are so many levels?
- Have you ever climbed a mountain?
- Why did Lolly climb the mountain?
- Are there mountains also inside of you that sometimes you feel you need to climb?

- Do you remember the first Goddesses' gift? What did Lolly do with this gift?
- Stones are usually found where? Would you say that a stone could be the beginning of a strong foundation?
- What colour was the stone?
- What did Lolly tell herself she wouldn't do at this point? (worry)
- Do you remember the second Goddesses' gift? What came out of the seed for Lolly?
- Did Lolly create the stairs or were they just automatically created? (no right answer)
- What colour was the seed?
- What did Lolly tell herself she wouldn't do at this point? (anger)
- What did the trees seem to be doing for Lolly along the way?
- What choice did Lolly make that suddenly made everything easier?
- Does that seem comparable to the flow of water with nothing in its way?
- Does paying attention help make things easier in your life?
- Lolly knew it wasn't going to be an easy climb, but what did she know she had to do to make it further?
- Why did Lolly get angry at her father and what did she say after she noticed her anger?
- What was on the wall that Lolly hit after she was guided by the trees?
- How come the path that Lolly was on had not been walked on before?
- What did the colour of the path seem to be?
- What were the animal images on the Map and which direction did they connect to?
- What two things did Lolly say to her mom when she entered the cavern?
- What colour of light did she see in the cavern?
- What happened to her as she found the right way through the cavern?
- What did she see along one wall?
- What was it used for?
- What did Lolly first see as she entered the fifth level?
- What did she have to do to move the vines?
- What did Lolly fall into?
- How did Lolly know she had found the healing energy that she could take back to her dad?
- How did she carry the healing energy back? How did she get back to her dad?
- Why do you think that she knew where to place her hands to help her dad?

- Is there a link to Lolly being able to heal with her hands and to her growing up to be so full of love!?
- How long did it actually take Lolly to learn all she needed to know?
- Do you think that it's possible that everything she learned was already within her and that she just needed to see it inside of herself?
- What did her father say that made everyone feel relieved and know that he was going to be all right?
- Do you think that you too can use the Emerald energy that Lolly gathered to help others like her father?
- Do you think you could also help yourself?
- Would you want to try this by using your hands too?
- Are you willing to put your hands in the Emerald Lake, just like Lolly, to gather the Emerald energy?
- Do you believe that the Emerald energy can also be used by you now, just like Lolly?
- Do you know that adults from around the world call the Emerald energy that you are using Reiki?
- Do you know that Lolly stated five practices throughout her journey that are commonly used by people who use the Reiki everyday? They are called the five Reiki principles. You can repeat them if you like. Do you remember during which parts of Lolly's journey she made these statements?

References

1   Rand, William Lee, <u>Reiki - The Healing Touch</u>, Vision Publications, Southfield, USA, 1991, pg 1-1.
2   King, Shirley, personal teachings, Ottawa, Canada, 2004.
3   Mirdad, Michael, <u>The Seven Initiations of the Spiritual Path</u>, A.R.E. Press, Virginia Beach, USA, 2004, pg. 18.

ABOUT THE AUTHOR

Cheryl Jiala Driskell is an Intuitive Energy Healer, Reiki Teacher and Program Director of an Anxiety and Depression, Intervention and Prevention program for Children and Youth, living in Ottawa, ON, Canada. Her years of studies in Sufism, Buddhism and Metaphysics have allowed her to see beyond what we believe to be true, as the stories' young adventurer will also soon discover.

Cheryl Jiala believes that it is only through love and acceptance that we can find a sense of personal peace and unity with all. Her dream is that this program be shared with Children and Youth everywhere, to assist them in forging a strong self awareness of their great potential in all ways, leading to personal empowerment and overall health. For more about Cheryl Jiala, please visit her website at www.jiala.ca.

6627045R00048

Printed in Great Britain
by Amazon.co.uk, Ltd.,
Marston Gate.